Walking for Beginners

Your Step by Step Guide for Hitting the Road!

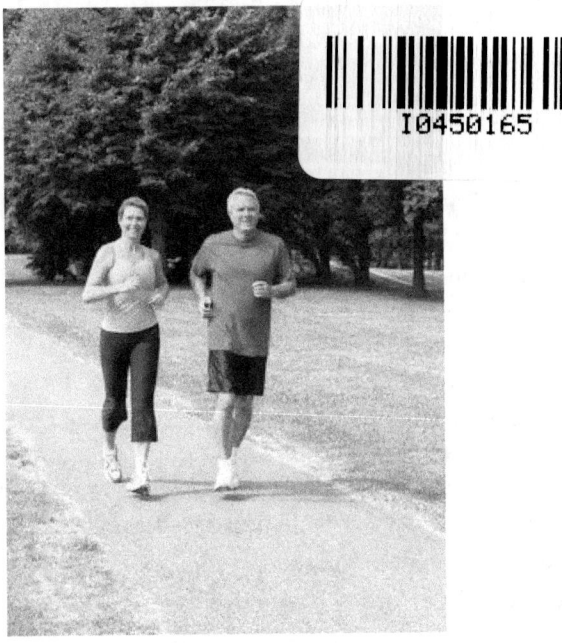

Health Learning Series

M. Usman

Mendon Cottage Books

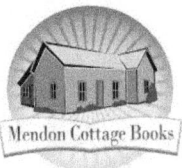

JD-Biz Publishing

Disclaimer

The information is this book is provided for informational purposes only. It is not intended to be used and medical advice or a substitute for proper medical treatment by a qualified health care provider. The information is believed to be accurate as presented based on research by the author.

The contents have not been evaluated by the U.S. Food and Drug Administration or any other Government or Health Organization and the contents in this book are not to be used to treat cure or prevent disease.

The author or publisher is not responsible for the use or safety of any diet, procedure or treatment mentioned in this book. The author or publisher is not responsible for errors or omissions that may exist.

Warning

The Book is for informational purposes only and before taking on any diet, treatment or medical procedure, it is recommended to consult with your primary health care provider.

Our books are available at

1. Amazon.com
2. Barnes and Noble
3. Itunes
4. Kobo
5. Smashwords
6. Google Play Books

Table of Contents

Preface

Walking - The word sounds so simple doesn't it? We perform the action every day and consider ourselves masters in it, but who knew that there might be a lot of things that aren't right when a person walks? Forget about the posture for a minute, walking is not just a way to go from one place to another, but also a wonderful technique to revive one's failing health and improving fitness. For perfect body health, however, it is necessary that a person walks with the right posture; moreover, there are variations with which he/she can walk and specific gear for maximizing the benefits.

This book will tell you about the correct procedure to walk, how to build up your schedule, and tell you all the requirements and must haves for a nice, good walk.

Walking Prerequisites

Chapter # 1: Medical Factors

Walking is a great natural way to achieve fitness, health, and the required amount of motion to initiate the process of weight loss. It is a wonderful way to maximize your physical activity throughout the day, which is never bad for you, and recommended by medical practitioners. Now, before the book puts you right to your feet, there are a few factors that must be considered by a person. It is necessary to contact a doctor for consultation before initiating the walking protocol as there might be a few things that aren't right with your body.

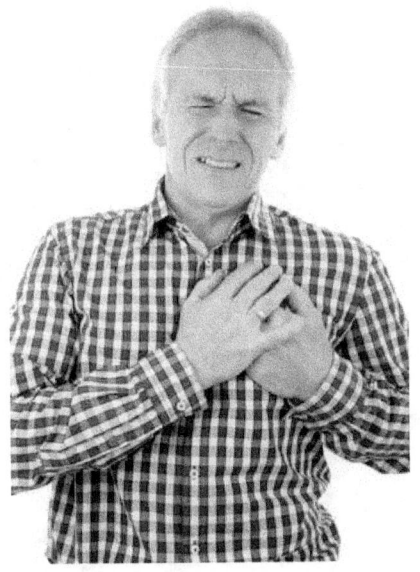

If you have any of the following medical signs or factors, you must contact your health care provider:

✓ Being sedentary or physically inactive for over a year. Too few people would think this applies to them, but the exact definition of being inactive states that it applies to a person who burns less than 1.5 kcal per kg of his/her body in a day. This could be converted into easier scales like 2 kilometers or 3000 steps.

- ✓   Being over the age of 65.

- ✓   Not indulging in any exercise, in addition to being over aged.

- ✓   You are pregnant.

- ✓   Your body is threatened by cardiovascular ailments.

- ✓   You have diabetes.

- ✓   You have recurring episodes of chest pain each time you physically exert yourself.

- ✓   Feeling faint.

Chapter # 2: Gear

You might think of walking as putting one step next to the other, but in reality it is more than just that. There are a number of factors that greatly motivate and boost up your mood when walking. These essential factors can make your experience more pleasant and can greatly lift your overall spirit, with respect to taking a walk. The following are the factors, necessary for a good, long walk.

> **Layered Clothing:** You may wear anything you like and go out for a walk, but maximum comfort and enjoyment can only be attained using layered clothing. By layering you ensure the body with having enough clothing for any condition. The fabrics chosen should be breathable and fine, so that they don't slow you down.

First, the base layer which are the clothes right next to the skin; the cloth you use as your base layer should be made of a fabric that draws sweat away from within your skin and not make you feel wet. Cotton is not the right type of cloth for this purpose as it does not release any sweat, it instead retains it. For cooler weather, look out for a material like polypropylene, while for warmer weather look for polyester fabrics.

Next, the insulating layer which is a must in colder weather; this layer is responsible for adding warmth to your body and is mobile to a level that it can be removed when you've warmed up. This should consist of pants or shirts made of fleece, pile, wool, or down. It is to be noted that you shouldn't wear too thick clothes for this layer as it can be daunting for you to walk after that.

Last is the outer layer that protects you from the elements, and can be removed as you warm up. The layer should be made up of windproof or water resistant fabric and be in the form of a jacket. For rainy days, look for fabrics that allow your body to breathe, but still keep the rain out like Ultrex. These fabrics may be more expensive, but you will surely notice the difference; a simple low grade fabric would make you as wet on the inside of your own sweat, as you are on the outside from the rain!

➢ **Shoes:** It is necessary to buy the right type of shoes for walking and not just go out in tap shoes, for all intents and purposes. There is a great variety of shoes, specially designed for different surfaces.

    i.   With regular athletic shoes, it is best to walk on asphalt surfaces as these give a bit as you walk, which reduces the impact of the foot.

    ii.   For pavements, try to get shoes with more cushioning as athletic shoes can tire your feet quite quickly on concrete.

    iii.   For rugged terrain, like dirt rocks or trails, pick harder shoes. Almost every brand of shoes that offers athletic shoes, also offers trail shoes. For walking, rather than backpacking, pick a lighter version with greater flexibility.

    iv.   In the rain, get a pair of water-proof shoes as there should be no excuse to break the cycle and routine that will be offered next.

    v.   For summers, buy a pair of rugged sandals as they will allow your feet to feel free.

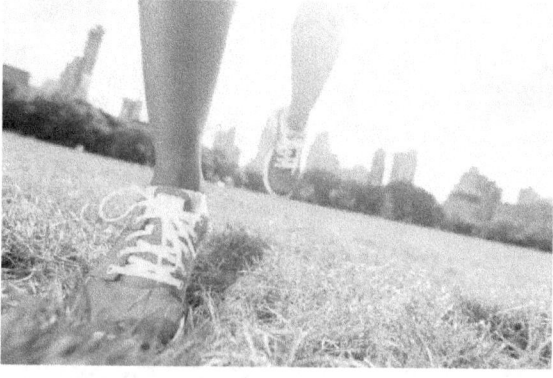

➢ **Socks:** That's right, every little detail is important, even the socks. Toss away the cotton tubes socks which will only cause discomfort in the form of blisters, and invest in pair or two of higher quality socks. Choose socks that are made of fabrics that help your sweat evaporate. Examples of these fabrics include, CoolMax, wicking fabrics, and polypropylene. Next, choose the ones with an ample amount of padding. The padding will keep you from getting tired when walking on the pavement; note that the padding will lower the impact, but require more room in your shoe. You may also buy double layered socks that consist of an inner sock made out of wicking fabric followed by an outer layer. These socks will deal with friction, sweat, and keep the blisters away. If the double layered socks are too expensive for you, make your own two layers by first wearing a sock made up of a wicking layer and the next one made out of wool.

Chapter # 3: Water

Water is must, before, during, and after a walk. Your stamina and level of comfort are greatly dependent on the amount of water you drink. You must drink every half hour, when walking at a normal pace, to restore the amount of fluid lost to perspiration. Let thirst be your guide though – do not fill yourself up with too much water that it starts bouncing around in your stomach. When going for long walks, plan your route in advance so that it contains a water spot. Have a good idea of the neighborhood or track so that you are aware of any water fountains that come on the way.

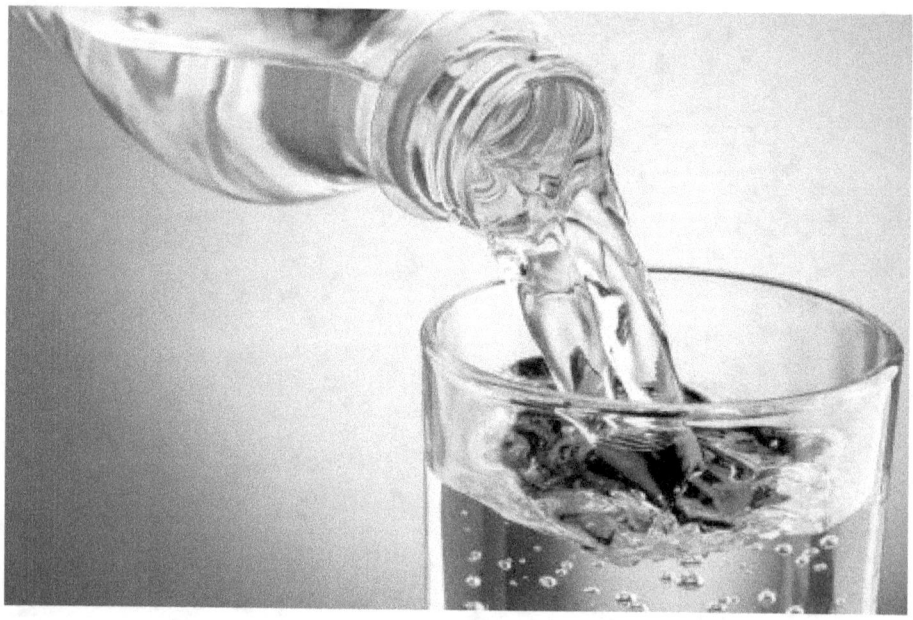

A pint or 500 ml per hour is necessary; and if you can get that from water fountains, then there is no need for a bottle. The best way to carry water, if you have to use a pack, is a backpack or a waist pack with an external bottle holder that can greatly help you get water quickly without any hassle. Otherwise, you may purchase a camelback which will allow you to carry water using the strength of your back and gulp it using a connected straw. Some waist packs have built in pouches for this purpose. Now, that you have the apparatus to carry a water bottle, it is time to decide on the water bottle. Visit a sporting shop and buy a good, reusable bottle with a wide mouth, so it can be easily cleaned, and ice cubes can be added to it. There are two varieties of water bottles generally available:

i.   Round

ii. Flat

The former one will fit easily in your packs; however look for a platypus shaped bottle which will stuff well in every pouch. Next, be sure of the water you carry. Never drink from an unsafe source before filtering and sterilizing it first. Don't try to pull a stunt like drinking from running sources, as these will most probably contain parasites and germs that can get into your liver and stomach and make you sick. Keep the bottle clean using soap; add a couple of drops of bleach overnight so it can be as clean as possible.

Chapter # 4: Optional Factors

If your outer layer is made up of sufficient amounts of pockets, then you may not need any type of pack. But, if you plan on becoming a hiker and walking from one town to the next, you might need a good pack to keep all your belongings. A good pack must evenly distribute the load on your back as well as your hips. There are a few options you may choose from depending on the length of your trip and the articles that you carry:

i. **Backpack** – A backpack is ideal for lengthy trips and bulky luggage as it gives you a lot of storage space, but it surely does reduce the comfort. Look for a backpack of the right size with a number of straps to take off the weight. An extra strap, known as belly strap, is necessary for larger back packs.

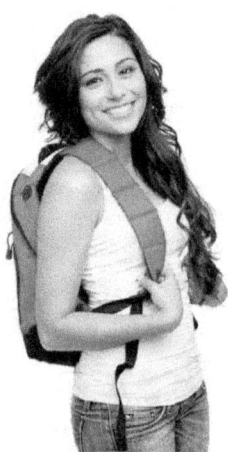

ii. **Waist pack** – Most normal walkers are satisfied with a medium sized waist-pack. Waist-packs are widely available in sporting shops and in a great number of varieties; try to look for a Waist pack that may hold your water bottle.

iii. **Hat** – A hat can prove to be a good companion on long sunny walks when the only thing between your head and the sun is the hat. A sun visor is the best choice when trying to improve your line of vision. A sun visor can keep the rays out of your eyes and provide a shade to the eyes. You may push your hair backwards if you want, which prevents excessive sweat from dripping outwards. Another choice when going for a walk is a general baseball cap. It keeps the sun off your face, shade in your eyes and also provides covering for your head. It also keeps any wind and rain off your head, and some caps even have inbuilt sweat padding that prevents excessive sweat from dripping. They also have a ponytail hole, just in case you plan on wearing one. These hats are multipurpose and may be used in all weathers; they have furthermore developed to such an extent that some even have LEDs and backlight strips for night time walking!

iv. **Walking wallet** – For a small routine walk, just pick a wallet for some identity documents and money. The wallet may not be of any specific type, but the regular one you take to work.

This may sound like something only women would do, but walking outside for lengthy periods of time can cause wrinkles, burns, and cancers so it is essential to get the right amount of protection, irrespective of gender:

i. Choose a sunscreen that is waterproof.

ii. Apply the sunscreen at least half an hour before walking.

iii. Put it on thickly and don't be shy – most people use too little of it and ultimately lack the protection they invested in.

iv. Apply it all over your face including ears.

v. Re-apply sunscreen if you perspire way too much.

vi. Apply a mosquito repellent if mosquitoes keep bugging you.

vii. Get anti-glare sunglasses that protect you from UVA and UVB.

These are pretty much all the factors that must be considered when going for a walk; all of them are not written in stone and you are free to adapt and choose them to your comfort. After all, it is your comfort that truly matters and making your own personalized combination is probably the best thing you can do.

Walking

Chapter # 1: Posture

Good posture is necessary for a soothing and comforting walk. It will allow you to breathe better and avoid many pains in and around your body, like back pain. The following are tips to a better posture when walking:

i.   First, stand up head held high.

ii.   Do not attempt to sit back, or lean back on your hips; this will only put strain on the back.

iii.   Do not arch your back; think as if you're tall and straight.

iv.   Some coaches many recommend that leaning at 5 degrees in the forward direction is great, but this is not good for beginners.

v.   Keep your eyes forward and try to look 20 feet ahead rather than below.

vi.   Relax your neck and don't hold your jaw with tension.

vii.   Get your chin parallel to the ground.

viii. Let your shoulders fall and position them slightly at the back; do not tense up your shoulders as this will increase strain on the body.

ix.   Suck in your stomach keeping the abdominal muscles straight and not over tightened.

x.   Rotate your hip in the forward direction which will help keep your back straight while keeping your head static as you walk.

You don't walk while keeping your arm stationary in space, they move along as you walk. This motion increases the amount of power transferred to walking by burning 5 – 10 % more calories. It balances your leg motion and gives you a natural look and not a robotic one. The following is the right way to move your arms while walking:

i.   Give your elbows 90 degree bend.

ii.   Don't tighten up your hands, rather given them a natural curl, not clenched and not fully open. Clenching would only raise your blood pressure which, as we all know, is not a good sign.

iii.   With each step, bring forward the arm that is opposite to your forward foot; it should up straight and not diagonal.

iv.   As one foot goes back, the other arm should now come forward while the first one should come straight back.

v.   Avoid flapping your arms, chicken winging, and high hands:

- What is meant by flapping arms? When a person doesn't bend his/her elbows, his straight arms flap like a bird or sometimes starts to paddle.

- What is chicken winging? When a person bends his/her elbows but swings them laterally, with one hand crossing past the central part of the chest; this actually endangers the pedestrians nearby.

- What are high hands? When you start to bring your shoulders up, higher than the normal limit that endangers your own nose.

vi.   The forward hand should not make a crossing at the central part of the body.

vii.   When coming forward, your hand should go as high as the breastbone.

viii.   If you find the prescribed arm motion tiring than carry it out for 5 – 10 minutes during each walk, not more.

Chapter # 2: Stepping

Walking a step is a simple rolling motion. To walk at a normal pace, feet will play a major role in the whole process rather than serving as launching and landing pads for the body. The body will make use of the heels and ankles to roll through each step and then finally push off, rather powerfully at the end of each stride.

i. The heel should hit the floor while the ankles should be flexed as the foot comes forward; think of it as trying to show people the front part of your shoe.

ii. When the foot lands, flex and roll through the step, starting from the heel and ending to the toe. The feet are designed to rotate in this manner, so you need not worry much. If your shoes are way too stiff, you would feel difficulty in rolling smoothly as you take each step. As the foot rolls, it actually passes under the whole body and carries the body's weight.

iii. The push you receive from the toe is the main supplier of force that raises your body. The push should only happen when your foot is positioned behind the body. As you push off via the foot positioned at the back, the opposite leg automatically comes forward to strike again.

iv. If the shoes you wear while walking are too stiff there will be two effects out of it. The first one would be the non-rolling motion of your feet as you take each step. The second would be more painful and give you aches as your shins would be fighting against your shoes to properly flex themselves.

v. As you begin to take faster steps, the shins of each leg will start to become more and sore and start developing shin splints. This is very common as it will still require a little time for your legs to get used to the right posture, and walking.

vi. While walking you should be sure that the ankle is doing the flexing each time your stride is in the forward direction and NOT the toes. If your toes start aching, it is a sign that the stride is not correct; therefore you will need to focus on your ankles instead.

vii.   The power as well as the developed speed should be coming from the rear leg and not the front one.

When practicing a stride, it is absolutely necessary that you keep over striding out of your system. This means taking longer steps to increase your speed. It is not only inefficient but also harmful as it increases the chances of getting an injury. Smaller steps, rather than lengthening your, stride are much better. Your stride should be longer behind the body, from where your toe pushes off. This is because the power for each step is derived from the back leg and not the front one. In order to get full power out of the back leg, the foot must be rolling from the heel to toe. Fast walkers must train themselves so as to increase the number of steps using their back leg.

Chapter # 3: Warming Up

Start out at a slow and easy pace before each session. Let your muscles warm up before you add speed, angle, or stretch to your walk. Warm up for at least 5 minutes at normal pace which won't make you breathe heavily. Stretching can greatly improve a person's flexibility, making the entire walk much more comfortable than before.

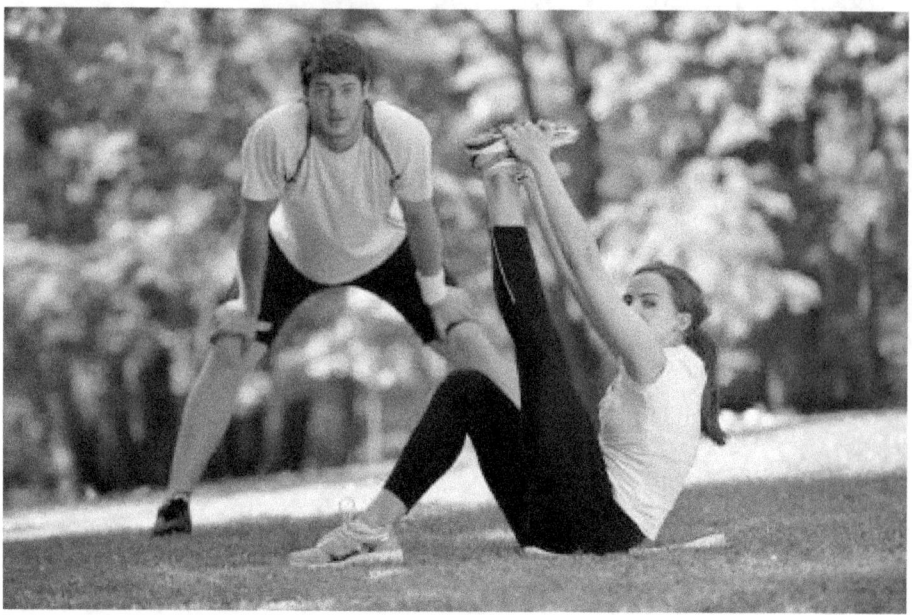

Never stretch cold muscles as this will only increase the risk of injury by tearing them apart. After ample warm up, start stretching by finding a fence, pole, wall, or anything with an upright structure to lean on. For walkers it is best to start with the following exercises:

i.   **Head circles:** The exercise starts at the top in order to loosen tension in the muscles in the neck which will help you with the correct posture and position. Note that your motions should be as smooth as possible when doing stretches; the procedure for a head circle is as follows:

•   Starting with your ear near your shoulder, rotate your head towards the front; continue to rotate with the other side as well, ending up at the ear which is near to the opposite shoulder.

- Repeat these steps; gently rotating your head at the other side.

- Repeat this 5 – 10 times.

ii.   **Arm circles:** To get ready for a good walking posture, loosen your shoulders along with the upper back using this exercise:

- Using one arm at a time, make a reverse arm circle with the palm facing out.

- Repeat this exercise 10 – 15 times.

- Now, make forward circles with the thumb pointed downwards.

- Repeat 10 times.

iii.   **Hip Stretch:** This particular stretch focuses on your hip muscles which are very much used in bringing the leg forwards:

- Stand up; place your right foot halfway back so that you are now in a lunge position.

- Bend the forward knee and shift your body to the right hip until a stretchy feeling comes on; keep a hold of this position for 10 seconds.

- While keeping the back leg straight, try to reach further down with the other leg; now try to hold this position for 30 seconds.

- Next, stand up and repeat the procedure with the other leg.

- Deepen the stretch as much as you can and hold the position for 30 seconds.

iv. **Quadriceps Stretch:** For this particular exercise, finding a wall or an upright post can be a source of easiness as it would involve finding stability using one foot. The exercise targets the quadriceps muscles that are used in activities like climbing or walking, etc.

- Stand straight and if possible get hold of a wall or pole.

- Bend your knee, (any knee) behind you in the air so that you are able to grab a hold of your foot; hold your heel against your butt and if you are trained enough, you may do this with the other hand on the side of the other leg.

- Stand up erect once again and push your knee as far as possible without putting much strain on it. Don't add any pressure using your hands.

- Keep at this position for 30 seconds before gently releasing your feet.

v. **Gastrocnemius Calf Stretch:** Stand at arm's length from a wall post and:

- Lean into the post, resting your palms on it.

- Place one leg forward and bend one knee as if no weight were on it.

- Keep the other leg back with the first knee straight and heel facing down.

- While keeping your back straight, move your hips towards the wall until a stretchy feeling appears.

- Hold at this spot for 30 seconds.

- Relax and repeat with the other leg.

vi. **Leg Extensions:** Have a wall at your side before doing this exercise to maintain your balance.

- Bend one of your knees while bringing one of your legs in the forward direction; extend it and swing the leg back and behind.

- Repeat these swings 15 times.

- Switch legs.

Next comes the process of walking, after which comes cooling down which is the last 10 – 15 minutes of your walk. Finish these minutes at a slower pace than before which allows you to let your body shed any heat that it built during the walk; it also returns your heart rate to normal. If you want, do the stretches you did earlier.

Chapter # 4: The Beginners Schedule

Walking for half an hour a day or approximately 3 hours a week is well associated with health benefits like the reduction in the risk of heart disease. Walking for 7 hours a week brings in even more perks with the reduced risk of breast cancer, and in some cases of type 2 diabetes. For this reason, it is essential that you keep on your feet for most part of the day. Walk at least 5 days in a week, even if you have to cut down on the average time spent walking; this is essential as it will help you in building a new habit.

Week # 1:

Start off with a 15 minute walk at a slow pace. Walk at least 5 days in the first week, as this is important to gain consistency. Spread out the rest days in between the walking days like make day 3 and day 6 the rest days.

Goal = 60 – 80 minutes

Week # 2:

Add five minutes to your walk each day so that compared to the first week you are walking 20 minutes a day for five days. If you want, you may add in more time; it's up to you now.

Goal = 80 – 100 minutes

Week # 3:

Add five minutes to the previous schedule so that now you are walking 25 minutes for 5 days.

Goal = 100 - 130 minutes

Week #4:

Add five minutes to the previous schedule so that now you are walking 30 minutes for 5 days.

Goal = 125 - 150 minutes

If you find the any week is difficult, repeat the week before and if you want, you may go through the cycle once again until you are bold enough to go on to higher workout schedules.

Chapter # 5: Mistakes while Walking

Walking in the right posture can greatly improve your fitness, health, and lifestyle, but in the wrong way, it won't do you any good. It is thus better to realize your mistakes and correct them before they become your habits. The first mistake that every person tends to make is over striding. People who try to walk faster damage their natural inclination by lengthening the stride at the front to reach out as far as possible using the forward foot. This results in an ungainly, clumsy walking posture that results in shin injury and honestly, you don't achieve that much speed. To cure over-striding you must understand that all the power comes from the back foot. Therefore, you must take shorter yet quicker steps if you want to achieve a greater pace. Also, be sure to roll through as you take each step which will provide you with a good push off.

There also might be some problem with your walking gear if you are uncomfortable during your walk. It should be well understood that not all walking shoes are designed for walking and thus shouldn't be walked in every time for a dedicated walk. The following are a few types of shoes that might create problems for you:

i.   **Heavy:** If the walking shoes add weight to your foot and you find it difficult to lift it off, you may want to switch to lightweight shoes.

ii.   **Over 1 year old:** The quality of the shoes starts to degrade as time passes so be sure to replace your shoes after walking 500 miles.

iii.   **Stiff:** If the shoes you wear are too tight and refuse to give in to the rolling motion of the foot, then maybe it's time to shift to something more flexible that will give your shin, as well as your foot, some relaxation.

You might be flat footed, which means walking with a flat foot instead of rolling from your heel to toe. If the foot is flattened pre-maturely it can seriously degrade your walking time. The best cure for this is to get as flexible shoes as possible, which will ensure that you get a bend from the ball of the foot. The best combo would be shoes with the least amount of heal. You may also do a few exercises to get your action right; one of these exercises involves standing on the stairs, facing upwards while your heels hang over the edge. Dip one of your heels downwards and then upwards; repeat this 10 – 15 times.

The motion of your arms is pretty much natural when it comes to walking, but some people either don't move their arms at all or swing them without giving it a bend. Arms are moved as you walk to act as counter balances, but keeping your arms stiff would not only make you look awkward but also give you a higher chance of falling off balance. Moreover, they will slow you down therefore move your arms effectively as they add speed as well as power to your motion.

People also tend to lean while walking, sometimes a little too much! Leaning is all right as long as it is 5 degrees in the forward direction. You may also lean back; somewhere you must have read that leaning forward while walking is good or leaning back on the hips can be useful. Both of these actions when performed excessively can cause back pain and make your posture worse. Stand up straight with relaxed shoulders with your chin parallel to the ground; suck in your gut, giving your back the natural curve it already has. Another way to prevent leaning is by strengthening the body's abdomen through sit ups which would result in a more complete look.

In the end, some people just lose it; they walk and keep walking until they lose all their motivation and feel tired of the whole procedure. The cure is simple; give yourself a break in the form of a rest day on which you don't walk. It allows the body to repair itself and also gets it motivated for the next day. Also make sure that you sleep normally as it really induces the best of the benefits of a workout. If you're trying to strengthen your body then you'll be glad to know that walking makes the muscles at the back the legs stronger; it makes the calves, gluteal muscles and hamstrings more durable which would help you maintain your balance, good posture, and health in general.

Conclusion

Did you ever think of a magic exercise being produced that would bless you with a decrease in the risk of major diseases like heart disease, diabetes and breast cancer? Well, there is an answer to this question now. Scientists have been astonished by studies which have shown remarkable effects on human health; the subject of these studies was none other than walking. That's right, walking can bring in a great number of health benefits for the body and not just ordinary ones, but the ones that protect you from life threatening diseases. It's simple; you strap on your shoes and start taking a walk. The results of a 20 year, lengthy Health Study have shown that brisk walking or waling in general can significantly reduce the risk of Type 2 diabetes, as well as breast cancer, in women. The way to achieve this goal has been explained in detail in the book and no stone has been left unturned in motivating you to change yourself. Walking can be a fun endeavor only if you want it to be so. If not, it will only tire and irritate you which will give you the least amount of satisfaction. Thus get yourself motivated as the mistakes and the preparations have all been highlighted; it's up to you now to follow them.

Best of luck!

References

http://www.fotolia.com/id/39676947

http://www.fotolia.com/id/41000500

http://nl.123rf.com/photo_15150282_loopschoenen-close-up-van-de-vrouw-op-blote-voeten-loopschoenen.html?term=shoes

http://nl.123rf.com/photo_21036145_stromende-water-uit-fles-in-glas-op-een-blauwe-achtergrond.html?term=water

http://nl.123rf.com/photo_20557528_jonge-gelukkig-student.html?term=backpack

http://nl.123rf.com/photo_15321363_jong-gezondheid-paar-stretching-oefening-ontspannen-en-opwarmen-na-het-joggen-en-actief-is-in-het-pa.html?term=warm%20up

Author Bio

Muhammad Usman is a distinguished medical graduate of Allama Iqbal medical college (AIMC). He is a professional writer who has been in the field for more than 4 years. During this time he has produced 10,000+ articles, blogs, and eBooks on various niches related to diseases, health, fitness, nutrition, and well-being. He is a regular contributor to several journals related to medicine and surgery. He is the editor of several journals and newspapers.

Check out some of the other JD-Biz Publishing books

Gardening Series on Amazon

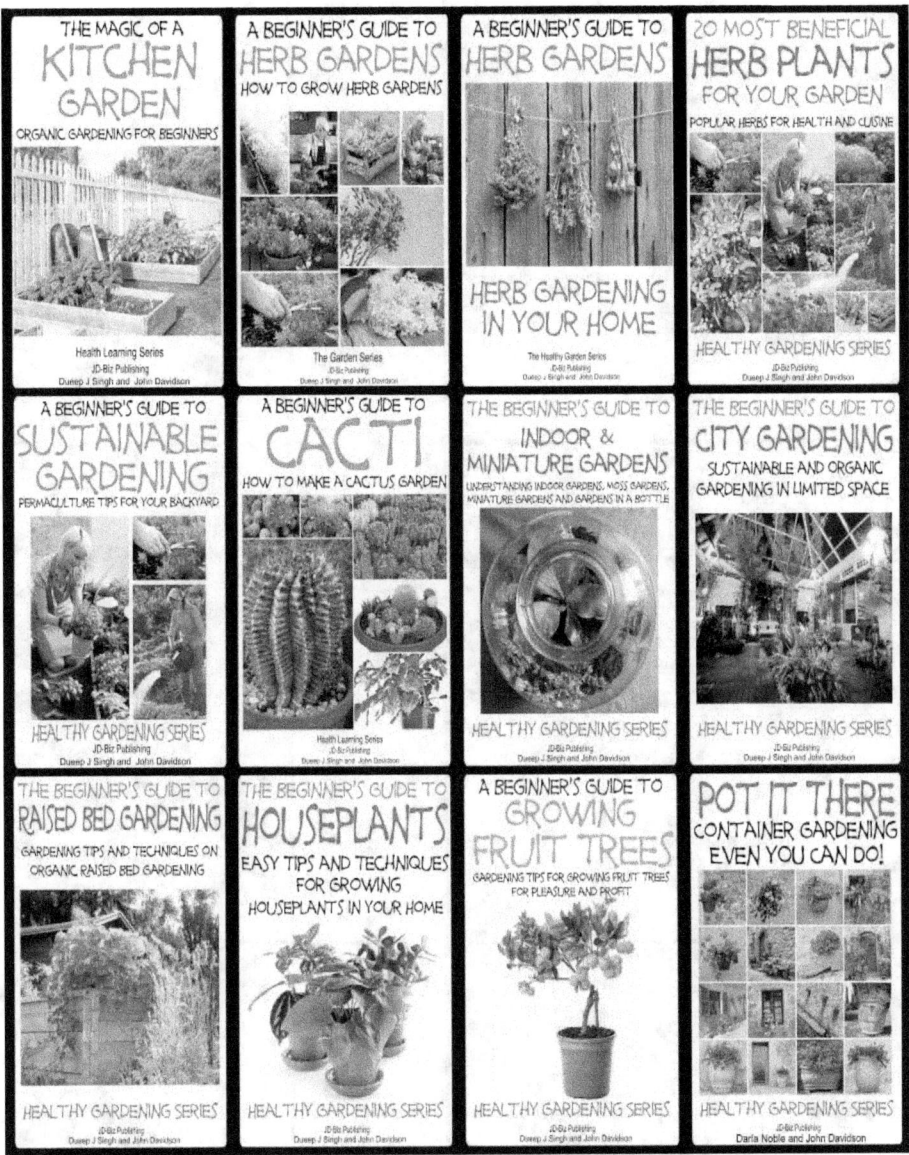

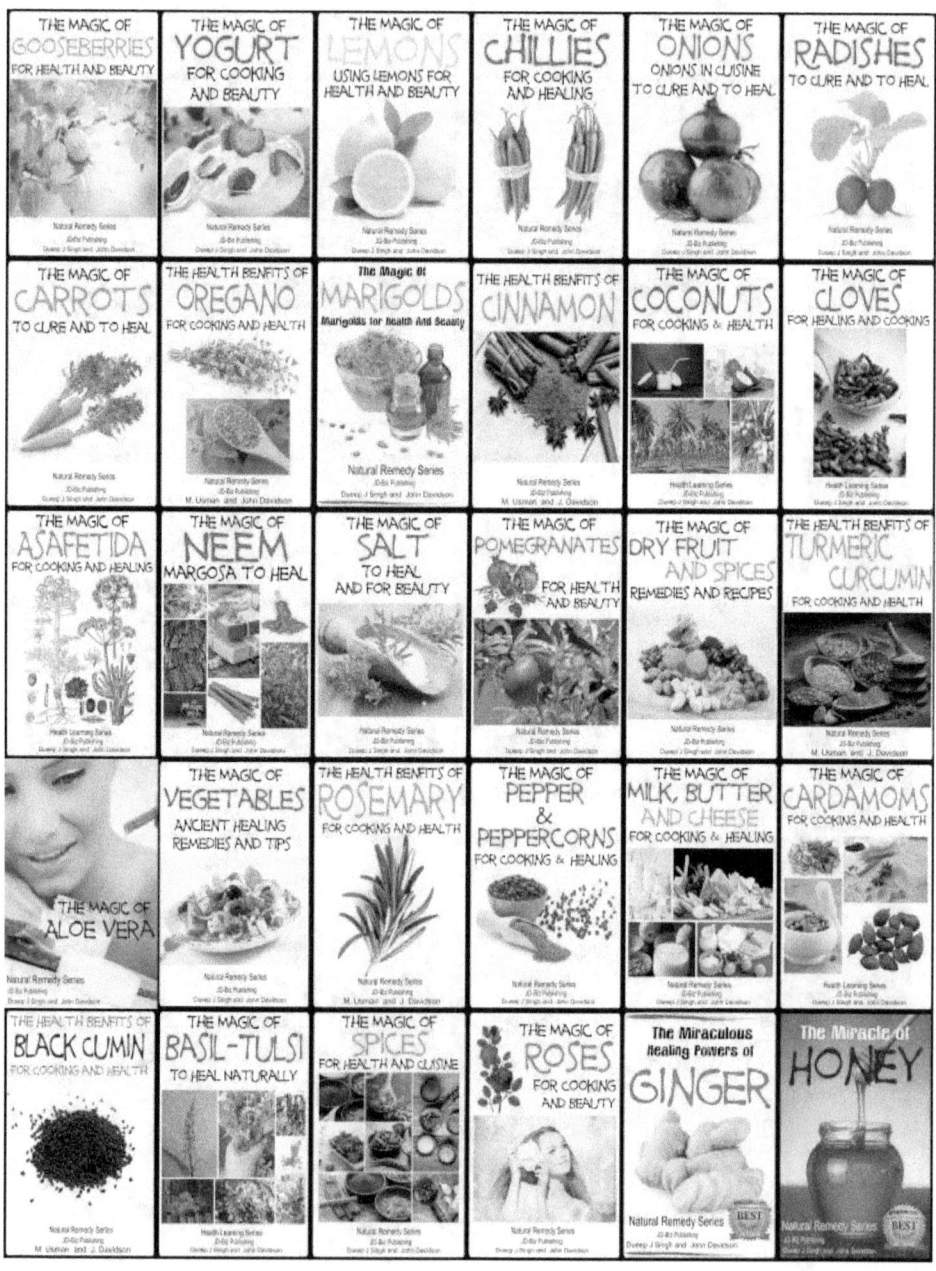

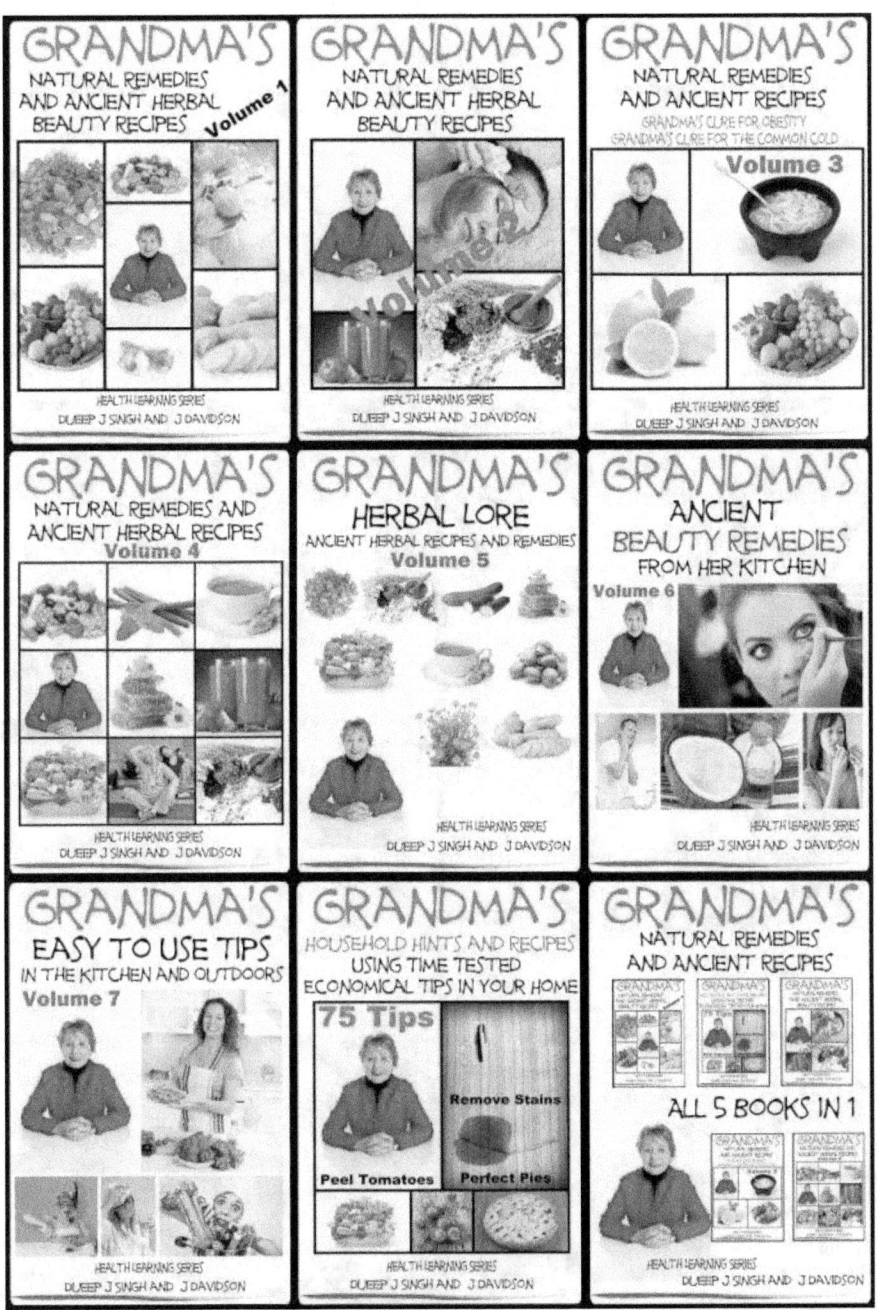

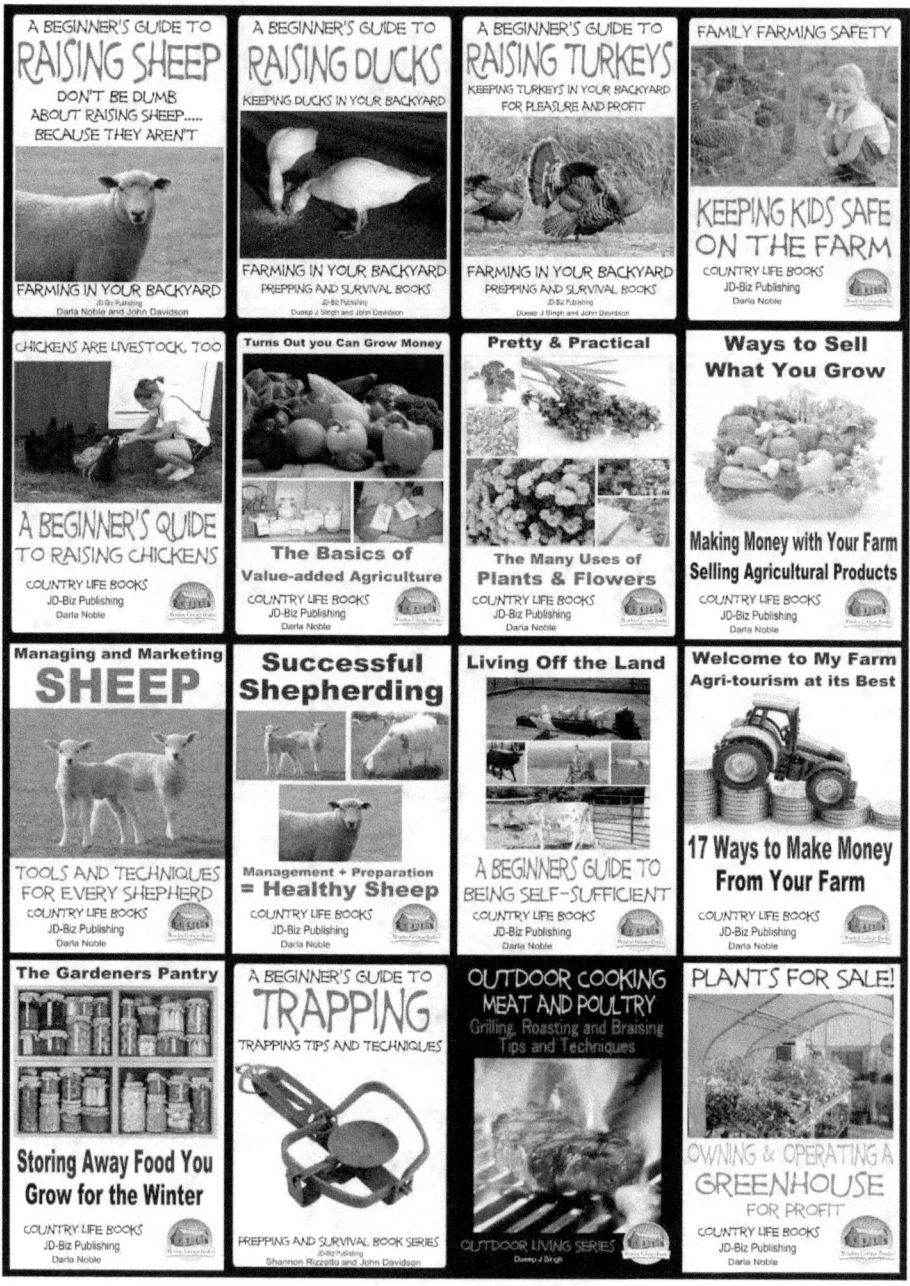

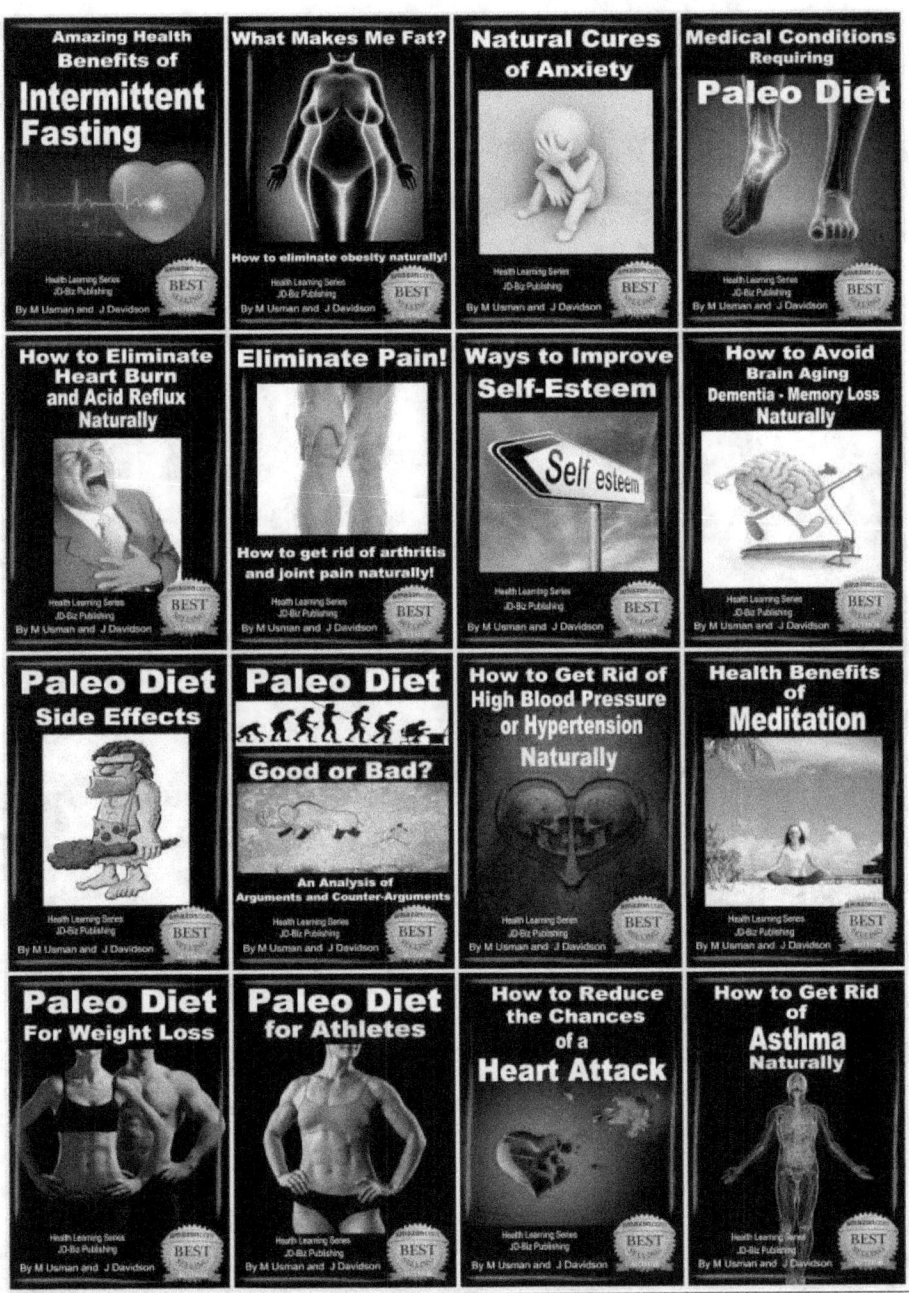

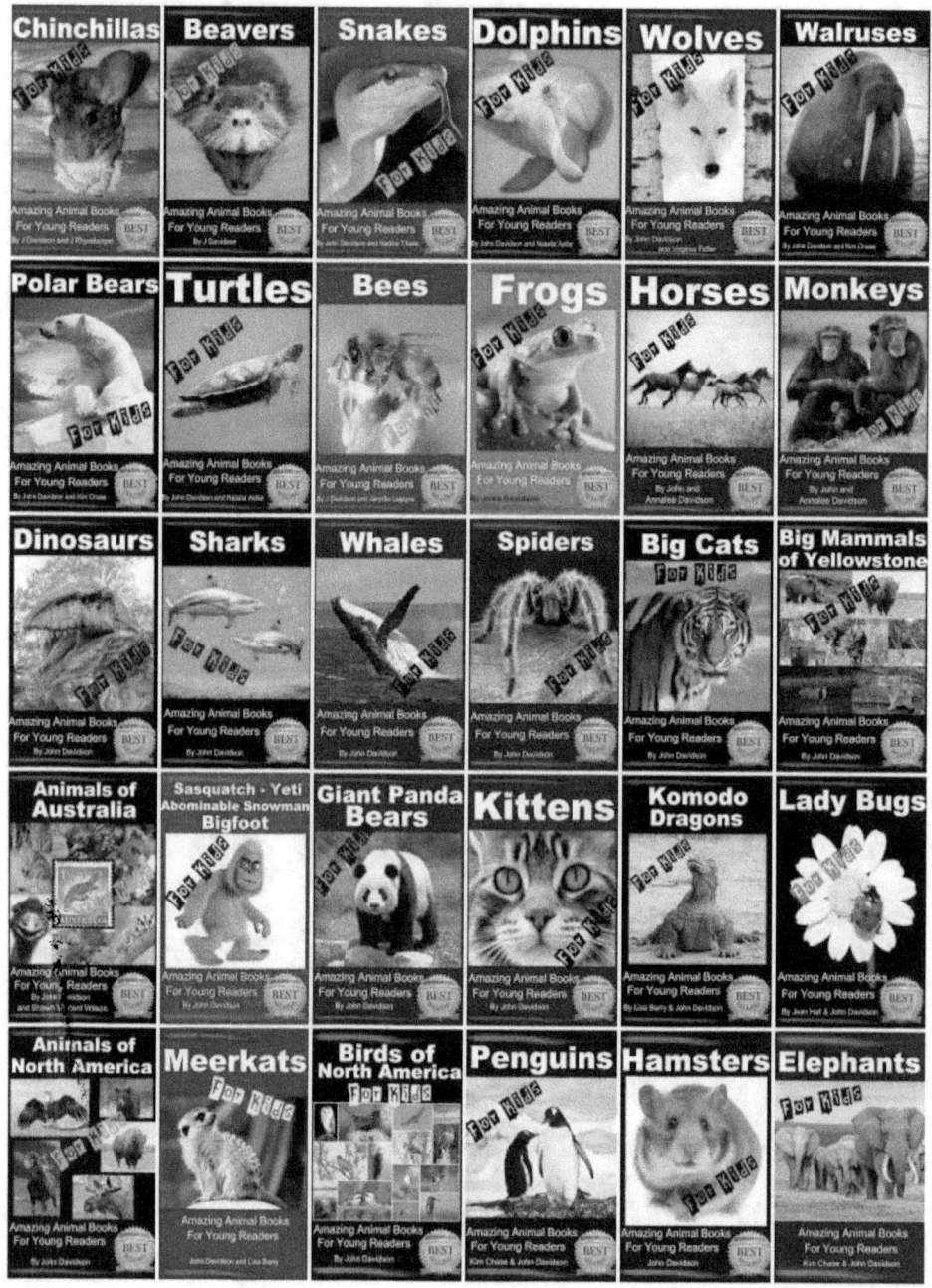

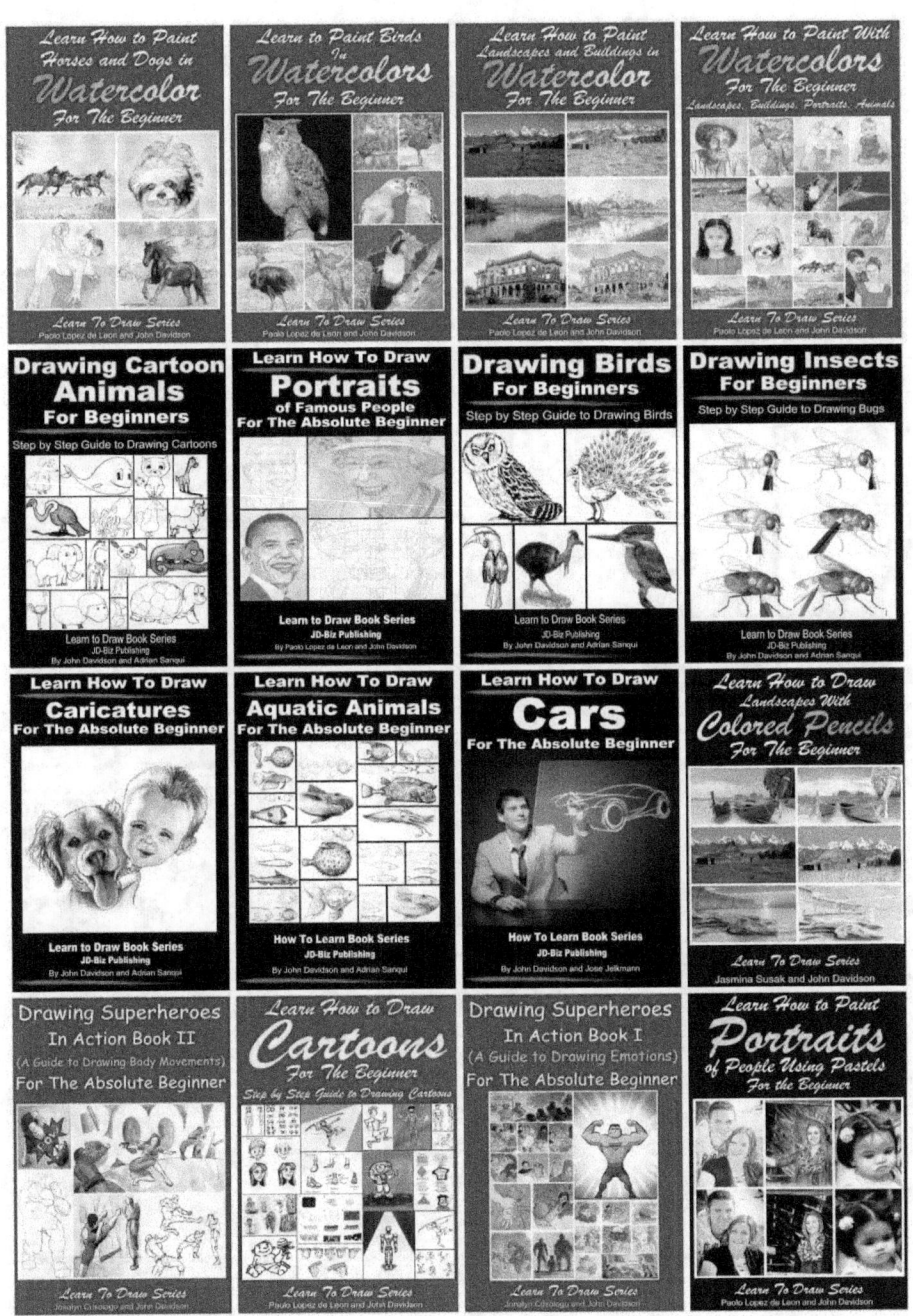

How to Build and Plan Books

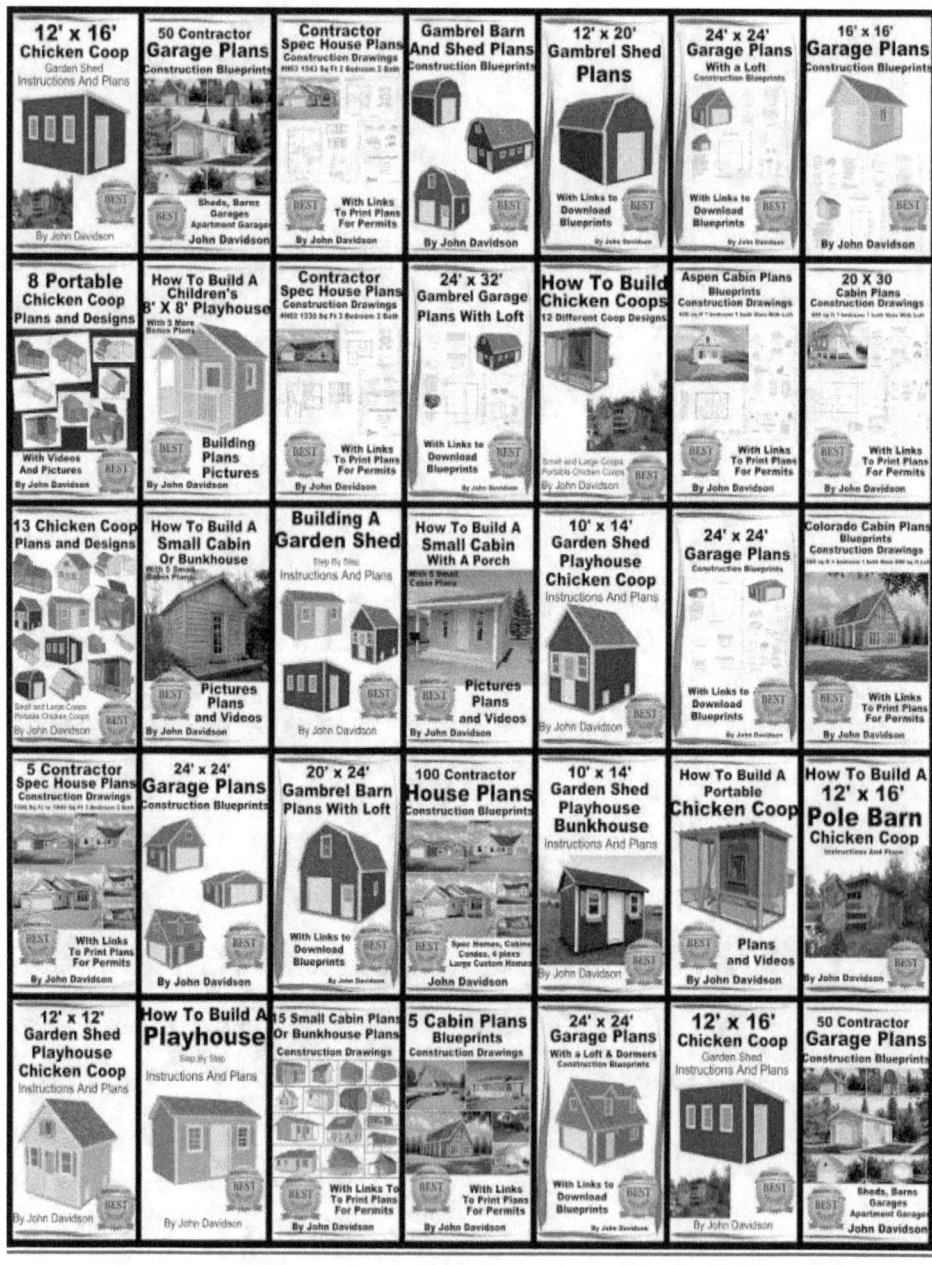

Entrepreneur Book Series

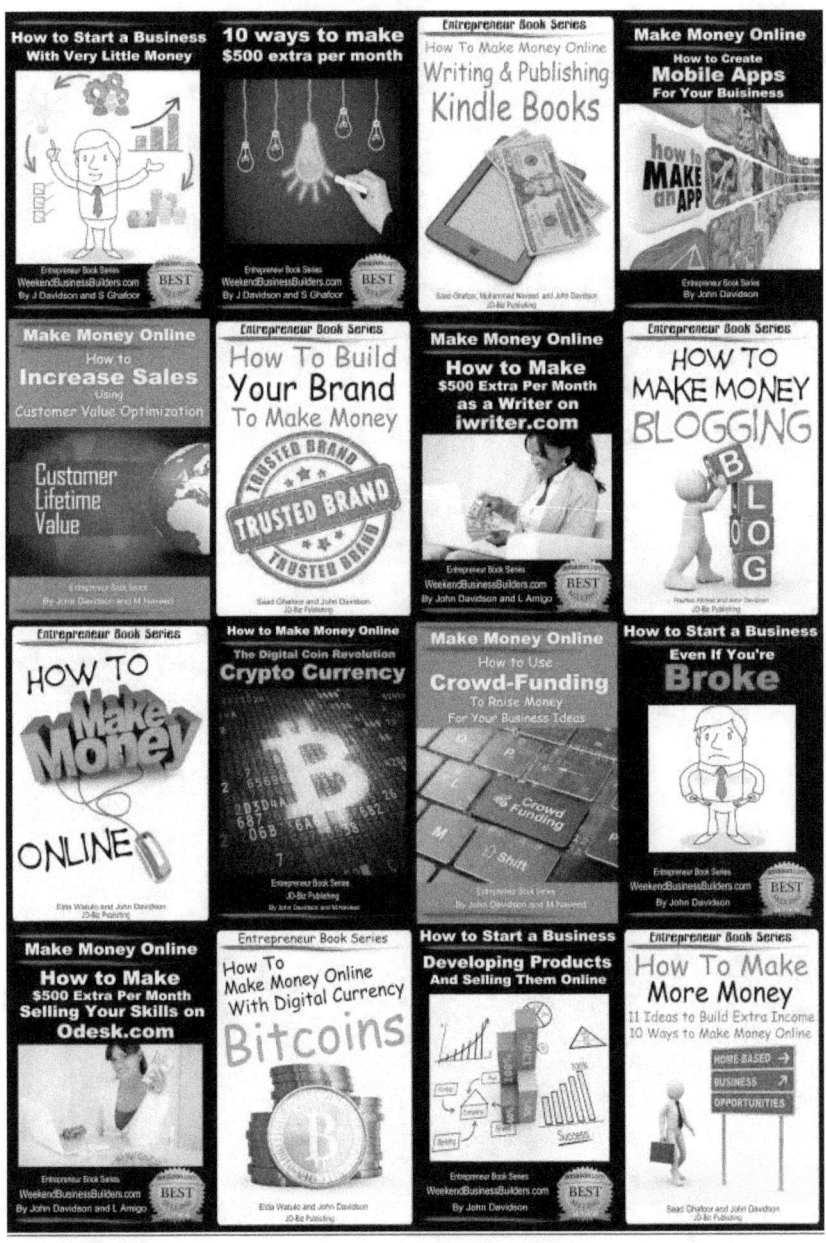

Our books are available at

1. Amazon.com

2. Barnes and Noble

3. Itunes

4. Kobo

5. Smashwords

6. Google Play Books

Publisher

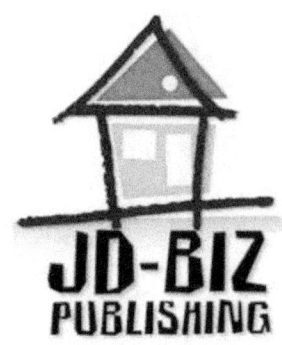

JD-Biz Corp

P O Box 374

Mendon, Utah 84325

http://www.jd-biz.com/

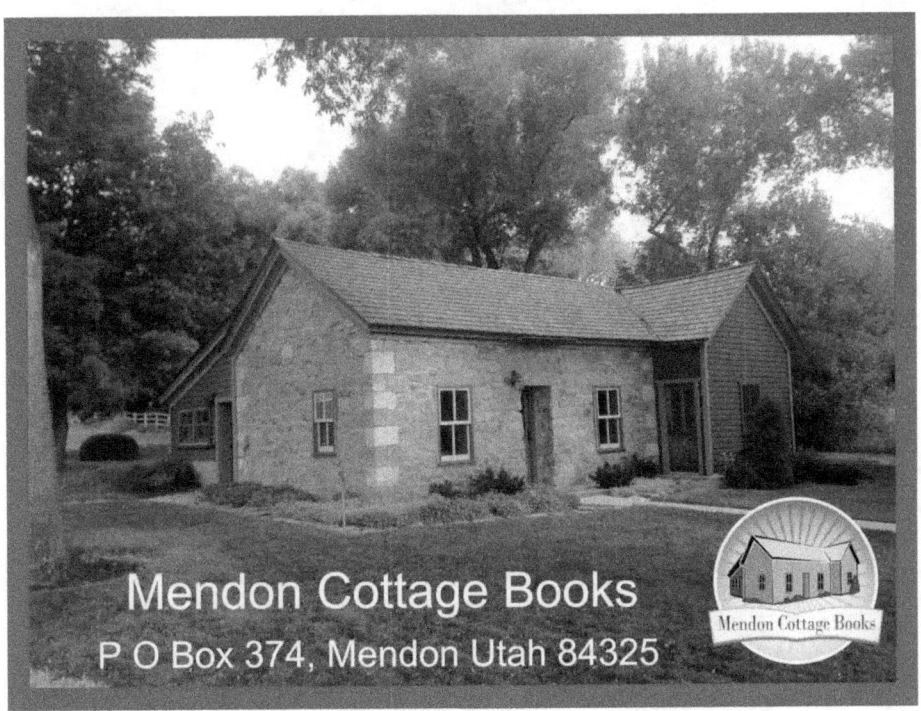

Mendon Cottage Books

P O Box 374, Mendon Utah 84325

www.ingramcontent.com/pod-product-compliance
Lightning Source LLC
Chambersburg PA
CBHW061932280526
45787CB00004B/1574